POCKET MANUAL TO CASE TAKING

POCKET MANUAL TO CASE TAKING

THIRD EDITION

Ravinder Nath Bansal
MBBS PGDMLS PGDHHM MPhil PhD
Deputy Medical Superitendent
GGS Medical College and Hospital
Baba Farid University of Health Sciences
Faridkot, Punjab, India

JAYPEE BROTHERS MEDICAL PUBLISHERS
The Health Sciences Publisher
New Delhi | London

Jaypee Brothers Medical Publishers (P) Ltd

Headquarters
EMCA House, 23/23-B Ansari Road,
Daryaganj New Delhi 110 002, India
Landline: +91-11-23272143,
+91-11-23272703
+91-11-23282021, +91-11-23245672
e-mail: jaypee@jaypeebrothers.com

Corporate Office
4838/24, Ansari Road,
Daryaganj New Delhi 110 002, India
Phone: +91-11-43574357
Fax: +91-11-43574314
e-mail: jaypee@jaypeebrothers.com

Overseas Office
JP Medical Ltd.
83, Victoria Street, London
SW1H 0HW (UK)
Phone: +44-20 3170 8910
e-mail: info@jpmedpub.com

EU GPSR Authorised Representative
Logos Europe, 9 rue Nicolas Poussin
17000, La Rochelle, France
Phone: +33 (0) 6 67 93 73 78
e-mail: contact@logoseurope.eu

Website: www.jaypeebrothers.com
Website: www.jaypeedigital.com

Pocket Manual to Case Taking
First Edition: 2001
Second Edition: 2003
Third Edition: 2018
Reprint: 2026
ISBN: 978-93-5270-399-9
Printed at: Samrat Offset Pvt. Ltd.

Preface to the Third Edition

Discipline is a must in every aspect of the life, which also holds true in medicine. Though taking and presenting a case in medicine is an art but it is also bound by certain rules. At one side is the sequence in which it has to be taken and on other side is the format for its presentation and recording of findings. Here in this book, an effort has been done to put this process in a simplified systematic manner. It is to be noted that everything in this book is point to point and readers are suggested to use it along with their standard detailed textbooks and also as per their teacher's guidance.

A lot of abbreviations have been used to keep the text to minimum trying to keep the book as concise as possible. Most of the abbreviations are self-explanatory and are commonly used.

Author is thankful to all of them who have directly or indirectly helped in bringing out this book. My special and sincere thanks to my friend Dr Ali Thahseen on whose computer this book took birth in year 2001, Dr Suhas Hydros for providing his valuable assistance and encouragement, Dr Sanjay Bhat, Dr Shibu Bahulayen, Dr Vivek Bansal, Dr Harshwardhan Gupta, Dr Sonu Gupta and Dr Amit Jindal for their kind help and to my teachers for their expert guidance, especially Dr VK Lekshmanan Kumar (Ex-Professor of Medicine, Medical College, Thrissur, Kerala).

Suggestions for the improvement and critical appraisal of the book from the readers are most welcome.

Ravinder Nath Bansal
E-mail: RNBansal@gmail.com

Preface to the First Edition

Discipline is a must in every aspect of the life, which also holds true in medicine. Though taking and presenting a case in medicine is an art but it is also bound by certain rules. One of which is the format in which it has to be taken and presented. Here in this book I have tried to put this process in a simplified systematic manner. I will like to make it clear that everything in it is point to point and readers are suggested to use it along with their standard detailed textbooks and also as per their teachers guidance.

I would like to thank all of them who have directly or indirectly helped me in bringing out this book.

I would like to thank my friend Dr Ali Thahseen on whose computer this book took birth and for the picture and formatting; Dr Suhas Hydros for providing his valuable assistance and encouragement to me; Dr Sanjay Bhat, Dr Shibu Bahulayen, Dr Vivek Bansal for their help and to my teachers for their guidance, especially Dr VK Lekshmanan Kumar (Professor of Medicine, Medical College, Trichur).

I welcome suggestions for the improvement and critical appraisal of the book from the readers.

Ravinder Nath Bansal

Contents

CHAPTER

1

Obstetrics Case Proforma

Name .... Age .... Address ....
W/o ....
Occupation ....
Socioeconomic status ....
Obstetric score: G....... P....... L........ A...............
LMP .... EDC ....
Gestational age .... weeks

PRESENTING COMPLAINT

....
....

HISTORY

History of Present Illness

- First visit to doctor
- Frequency of visits
- TT injections

Ist Trimester

- Morning sickness
- Bleeding/discharge PV
- Abdominal pain
- UTI (burning micturition/dysuria)
- Tiredness/fatigue
- Excessive salivation
- Iron and folic acid intake
- Drug intake, X-ray, fever (rubella, TORCH)
- Weight gain per week.

IInd Trimester

- Bleeding/discharge per vaginal (PV)
- UTI (burning micturition/dysuria)
- Edema—relieved by rest/not
- Quickening—which week
- Abdominal pain
- Hypertension (headache)
- Sudden increase/decrease in weight
- Iron and folic acid intake
- Drug intake, X-ray, fever, rubella
- Ultrasound.

IIIrd Trimester

- Bleeding/discharge PV
- UTI (burning micturition/dysuria)
- Edema—relieved by rest/not
- Fetal movements Y/N
- Hypertension (headache)
- Sudden increase/decrease in weight
- Iron and folic acid intake
- Drug intake, X-ray, fever, rubella.

Menstrual History

- Menarche, periodicity (e.g.—4/28)
- Menorrhagia/dysmenorrhea
- LMP.

Marital and Obstetric History

- Age at marriage
- Consanguineous Y/N
- Any period of infertility (any trt.)
- Any contraceptive use
- Previous children
  - Age at present
  - Weight at birth
  - Term/preterm
  - Associated complications (DM, PIH)
  - Any congenital anomalies.

Past History

- Polio, rickets
- Diabetes, hypertension, rheumatic fever
- Jaundice
- Surgery.

Personal History

- Sleep, appetite, addiction
- Bowel, bladder.

Family History

- Congenital anomalies, diabetes
- Hypertension, multiple pregnancy.

GENERAL EXAMINATION

- Ht…………, Wt………………
- Gait, breast, thyroid
- Built and nourishment
- Pallor
- Cyanosis, clubbing, jaundice
- Edema: Site _____leg/medial malleolus
- Lymphadenopathy
- Jugular venous pressure (JVP)

- Vital signs:
  - Pulse—rate, rhythm, volume, character, peripheral pulses
  - BP in right upper arm in supine position
  - Respiratory rate
  - Temperature (98.4°F).

OBSTETRIC EXAMINATION

Inspection

- Abdomen transversely/longitudinally distended
- Flanks full Y/N
- Any undue distention
- Striae gravidarum
- Linea nigra
- Umbilicus everted/not.

Palpation

- Quantity of liquor
- Fundal height—do not mention in cm—say FH corresponds to ……… weeks of gestation with flanks full/not
- Fundal grip
- Umbilical grip
- 1st pelvic grip
- 2nd pelvic grip
- Ballotment.

Percussion (do not mention, only few teachers may ask)

- Adequacy of amniotic fluid.

Auscultation

- Fetal heart:
  - Site
  - Rate
  - Rhythm.

DIAGNOSIS

Age, gravid, gestational age, coming with............ presentation in..........position. Head engaged/not and........complicating pregnancy.

CHAPTER

2

Pediatric Case Proforma

Name ...., Age ...., Sex ....
Address ....
Informant ....

PRESENTING COMPLAINT

....
....

HISTORY

History of Present Illness

Onset, progress, present status

History of Past Illness

- Similar illness
- Measles, mumps, whooping cough, TB, jaundice and hepatitis
- Surgeries.

Antenatal History

Ist Trimester

- Drugs
- Infection (TORCH)
- Radiation
- Trauma
- Checks ups (yes/no/regularity).

IInd Trimester

- APH, PIH, DM, HT, IUGR
- Jaundice
- Fetal movements
- Immunization
- Nutrition.

IIIrd Trimester

- APH, PIH, PPH, DM, HT, IUGR
- Jaundice
- Fetal movements
- Immunization
- Nutrition.

Natal History

- Term/preterm
- Hospital/home
- Vaginal/instrumental/cesarean
- Prolonged/normal labor
- Intranatal complications (if any)
- Baby cried immediately after birth/not
- Birth weight.

Neonatal History

- Umbilical sepsis
- Meconium: When passed
- Jaundice
- Dyspnea
- Feeding problem
- Seizures →
  - Day 1 → Trauma
  - Day 2 → Metabolic disorder
  - Day 3 → Infection (e.g. meningitis).

Developmental History

Gross Motor (It is Cephalocaudal)

Months	
04	Neck steadiness
05	Turning over
06	Sit with support
09	Sit without support
10	Stand with support
11	Stand without support
12	Walk with support
16	Walk without support

Fine Motor/Adaptive

Months	
1.5	Eye fixation
05	Mouthing
07	Single hand approach
09	Pincer grasp
12	Stops mouthing

Personal /Social

Months	
03	Social smile
04	Anxiety to strangers
15	Dry by day
2–2.5 years	Dry by night
3 years	Playing with children

Language

02 months	Alert to sounds
10 months	Monosyllables (mama)
1 year	3 meaning-full words
2 years	Few sentences

Dietetic History

- Breastfeeding (Y/N), how long
- Weaning
  - When started?
  - With what?
  - Any problems?
- Normal food, when given?
- Calculate calorie–protein intake.

Immunization History

• Birth	OPV (0), BCG, HepB
• 1 ½ months	OPV (1), DPT (1), HepB, Hib
• 2 ½ months	OPV (2), DPT (2), HepB, Hib
• 3 ½ months	OPV (3), DPT (3), HepB, Hib
• 9 months	Measles, JE
• 15 months	MMR (Measles, mumps and rubella)

- 1½ years OPV, DPT, JE, measles
- 5 years DPT
- 10 years TT
- 16 years TT

Note: Pentavalent = DPT + HepB + Hib

* JE and pentavalent — in select states only.

Family History

- Consanguineous marriage
- Any illness running in family
- History of tuberculosis
- Age of mother and father at marriage
- Age of mother at childbirth
- Congenital abnormalities
- Miscarriage, stillbirths, childhood death(s).

Socioeconomic Status

- Status: Poor/middle/high
- Working/not
- Whether mother separated from child.

Treatment History

GENERAL EXAMINATION

- ***General Survey***
  - Attitude
  - Built and nourishment
  - Height/weight
  - General examination
  - Vital signs.
- ***Head-to-foot Examination***
  - Head—size/shape, sutures, fontanelle, hair
  - Facies—eyes, nose, ears, mouth and lips
  - Teeth, palate, tonsil
  - Neck
  - Chest
  - Abdomen
  - Limbs
  - Spine.

Anthropometry

- Height
- Weight
- Head circumference
- Chest circumference
- Mid arm circumference
- Upper segment/lower segment ratio.

SYSTEMIC EXAMINATION

- Respiratory system
- Cardiovascular system
- Gastrointestinal system
- Nervous system.

DIAGNOSIS

Nutritional values

Item	*Quantity*	*Cals*	*Protein (g)*
Cooked rice 1 cup	200 g	175	4
Cooked daal	1 tsp	8	0.5
Sambhar	15 mL	45	0.75
Coffee milk 1 cup	150 mL	45	1
Cow's milk 1 glass	200 mL	130	7
Idli 1	40 g	100	3
Dosa 1	30 g	80	2
Chapati 1	40 g	100	3
Green leafy vegetable	100 g	--	4
EEG	50 g	80	6
Bread 1 slice	25 g	50	2
Vada 1	25 g	75	2.5
Bonda 1		50	1
Uppma 1 cup		250	6
Pappadam 1		20	0.5
Biscuit galaxo 1		20	0.5
Fish 4" × 5"	30 g	80	6
Groundnut	50 nos	100	5
.			
.			
.			
.			

Note: Add to list as per your need

RDA of vitamins (Approximate values)

Vitamin	*Infant*	*Child*	*Adult*
A	400 IU	400 IU	750 IU
C		20 mg	40 mg
D	200 IU	400 IU	400 IU
B_1 thiamin		0.5 mg	1 mg
B_2 riboflavin		1 mg	2 mg
Nicotinic acid	10 mg	10 mg	20 mg
Pyridoxine	1 mg	2 mg	2 mg
Folic acid	0.1 mg	0.1 mg	0.2 mg
B_{12}	0.001 mg	0.001 mg	0.002 mg

Calorie Requirement per Day

Up to 6 months	120 kcal/kg/day
7–12 months	100 kcal/kg/day
1 year	1000 kcal/day
>1 year	1000 + (small age–1) × 100 kcal/day

Protein Requirement per Day

<3 months	2.25 g/kg
3–12 months	1.75 g/kg
1–6 years	1.5 g/kg

CHAPTER

3

Respiratory System Case Proforma

Name ...., Age ...., Sex ....
Address ....
Occupation ....
Socioeconomic status ....
Date of admission ....

PRESENTING COMPLAINT

....

....

HISTORY

History of Present Illness

- *Cough*
  - Onset, duration, progress
  - Episodes
  - Expectoration
  - Aggravating factors—seasonal, diurnal, postural
  - Relieving factors—rest, drugs.

- *Expectoration*
  - Onset, duration, progress
  - Quantity—scanty/copious
  - Amount ____ mL/day, ______cups/day
  - Variation → diurnal, seasonal, postural
  - Color
  - Consistency
  - Foul smelling
  - Blood stained.
- *Hemoptysis*
  - Onset
  - Duration
  - Progress
  - Quantity, frequency of episodes
  - Fresh/altered.
- *Breathlessness*
  - Onset, duration, progress
  - Dyspnea — Grade....(1–4)
  - Orthopnea
  - Paroxysmal nocturnal dyspnea (PND)
  - Aggravating factors, relieving factors.

- *Chest pain*
  - Onset
  - Duration
  - Progress, episodes
  - Site, type, lasting
  - Radiation
  - Aggravating factor….respiration
  - Relieving factor
  - Associated night sweats.
- *Wheezing*
  - Onset, duration
  - Progress—constant/intermittent
  - Inspiratory/expiratory
  - Aggravating factors—seasonal, diurnal, postural
  - Relieving factors—rest, drugs
  - Associated skin rashes
  - Dust, food allergy.
- *Fever*
  - Onset
  - Duration
  - Type
  - Associated chills and rigors
  - Diurnal variation
  - Night sweats.

- *Rule out sinusitis*
  - History of nasal discharge
  - History of headache
  - History of recurrent cold
  - History of allergy to dust, pollen, etc
  - History of ear pain/discharge.
- *Rule out tuberculosis*
  - Cough with expectoration
  - Anorexia (duration)
  - Weakness
  - Weight loss (how much)
  - Low-grade fever with evening rise of temperature
  - Hemoptysis.
- *Rule out mechanical compression*
  - Dysphagia
  - Hoarseness of voice
  - Breathlessness
  - Puffiness of face
- *Rule out CNS involvement*
  - Seizures
  - Facial asymmetry
  - Peripheral neuropathy
  - Cerebellar signs

- *Rule out CVS involvement*
  - Edema
  - Palpitation
  - Syncope.
- *Rule out renal causes*
  - Swelling of face
  - Oliguria
  - Color of urine.
- *Rule out abdominal causes*
  - Abdominal pain
  - Jaundice
  - Dysphagia
  - Diarrhea
  - Vomiting
  - Hiccups
  - Abdominal distension.

Past History

- Similar illness
- TB, DM, IHD, asthma, jaundice
- Childhood illness—whooping cough, measles, influenza.

Family History

- Similar History of DM, TB, HT, IHD
- Parents marriage consanguineous
- Asthma, eczema.

Personal History

- Appetite
- Veg/Non-veg
- Bowel
- Bladder
- Alcohol—amount, duration
- Smoking—no(s), duration
- Sleep.

Menstrual History

- Menarche, LMP
- Regular, amount [no(s) of pads used]
- Associated pain.

Treatment History

From where, duration.

GENERAL EXAMINATION

- Built and nourishment
- Conscious and cooperative
- Pallor, cyanosis, clubbing, jaundice
- Edema
  - Site—leg/medial malleolus
  - Pitting/nonpitting
  - Unilateral/bilateral
  - Sacral, facial.
- Lymphadenopathy
  - Site
  - Temperature, tenderness
  - Size, no(s), shape, surface
  - Consistency
  - Mobility/fixity, matted
  - Discharge.
- JVP
- Vital signs
  - Pulse—rate, rhythm, volume, character, vessel wall, R-F delay, peripheral pulses
  - BP in right upper arm in supine position
  - Respiration—rate, type (thoracoabdominal)
  - Temperature (98.4°F).

RESPIRATORY SYSTEM EXAMINATION

Respiratory rate = .../ min

Upper Respiratory Tract

- Flaring of nose
- DNS
- Throat
- Tonsils
- Sinus tenderness.

Lower Respiratory Tract

Inspection

- Shape: Normal/barrel/flattened
- Bilateral movement (equal/not)
- Subcoastal angle: Normal (70°)/widened
- Dyspnea (intercostal withdrawing)
- Accessory muscles (involved/not)
- Trachea: Position
- Trail's sign
- Apex beat visible in ....

- Suprascapular hollowing
- Infraclavicular flattening
- Suprascapular wasting
- Shoulder drooping
- Spine: Kyphosis/scoliosis/lordosis
- Visible scars/dilated veins/sinuses
- Chest expansion ...cm (normal = 3–6 cm)
- Hemithorax ....(cm)
- Movements: Normal and equal/ decreased in .... area.

Palpation

- Temperature (equal/unequal) on both sides
- Local rise of temperature (if any)
- Trachea central
- Apex position
- Rib crowding (+/-)
- No...bony tenderness
- Vocal fremitis (compare all areas of both sides)
- No palpable rub, rhonchi, rales.

Percussion

- Resonant/impaired/dull in right/left.
  - Supraclavicular/clavicular/infraclavicular area
  - Mammary area
  - Axillary/infra-axillary area
  - Suprascapular/interscapular/infrascapsular area.
- Upper border of liver
- Tidal percussion
- Shifting dullness
- Traube's area (normally resonant).

Auscultation

- Compare bilaterally and over all areas separately
  - Intensity of breath sounds (↑, ±, ↓)
  - Character of breath sounds
  - Vesicular/bronchial (Tubular/amphoric cavernous)
  - Adventitious sounds—crepitations/rhonchi (area)
  - Vocal resonance ↑, ±, ↓ (areas)
  - Coin test—hydropneumothorax
  - Succussion splash.

ABDOMEN

- Hepatomegaly
- Splenomegaly
- Ascites.

CARDIOVASCULAR SYSTEM

- Apex beat .... displaced/not
- S1, S2 normally heard.

CENTRAL NERVOUS SYSTEM

- No facial abnormality
- All reflexes are normal.

DIAGNOSIS

- Bilateral/unilateral
- Ranchi/wheeze/creps
- Bronchial breathing (area)
- Pleural effusion
- Hydropneumothorax
- Probably due to TB/post TB/infection/pneumonia.

CHAPTER

4

Cardiovascular System Case Proforma

Name ...., Age ...., Sex ....
Address ...., Occupation ....
Socioeconomic status ....
Date of admission ....

PRESENTING COMPLAINT

....
....

HISTORY

History of Present Illness

- *Chest pain*
  - Onset
  - Duration
  - Progress, episodes
  - Site, type, lasting
  - Radiation

  - Associated sweating, syncope, discomfort
  - Aggravating factor (respiration/exertion)
  - Relieving factor (drugs/rest).
- *Palpitation*
  - At rest/exertional
  - Onset
  - Progress
  - Duration
  - Paroxysmal (+/-)
  - Relieving factors (rest/drugs)
  - Aggravating factors (exertion/straining).
- *Breathlessness*
  - Onset
  - Duration
  - Progress
  - Grade (1–4)
  - Orthopnea/PND
  - Aggravating/relieving factors.
- *Cough*
  - Onset, duration, progress
  - Episodes
  - Expectoration
  - Aggravating factors (seasonal, diurnal, postural)
  - Relieving factors (rest drugs).

- *Expectoration*
  - Onset, duration, progress
  - Quantity—scanty/copious
  - Amount ..... mL/day (or) ...... cups/day
  - Color
  - Consistency
  - Foul smelling (+/-)
  - Blood stained (+/-)
  - Aggravating factors—seasonal, postural, diurnal
  - Relieving factors—rest/drug.
- *Blood in sputum*
  - Onset
  - Duration
  - Progress
  - Episodes [No(s). and amount]
  - Fresh/altered
  - Aggravating factors
  - Relieving factors.
- *Syncopal attacks*
  - Onset
  - Duration
  - Progress
  - Episodes, lasting

- Aggravating factors
- Relieving factors.

- *Convulsions*
  - Onset, duration, progress
  - Episodes
  - Aggravating factors and relieving factors
  - Associated fever
  - Any froth/tongue biting
  - Whole body/one part
  - Loss of consciousness and for how long.
- *Rule out CCF*
  - Anorexia, nausea, vomiting
  - Right hypochondrial pain
  - Pedal edema
  - Breathlessness.
- *History suggestive of thromboembolism*
  - History of hemiplegia
  - Limb weakness, muscle cramps/pain
  - Any major surgery in recent past
  - Prolonged immobilization
- *Rule out rheumatic heart disease*
  - Fever with sore throat
  - Fleeting joint pains
  - History of 3 weekly injections
  - Valvular disease.

- *Rule out infective endocarditis*
  - Fever high grade
  - Progressive pallor
  - Hemiplegia
  - Complications of infective endocarditis.
- *Rule out congenital heart disease*
  - Cyanotic/acyanotic
  - Failure to cry immediately after birth
  - Failure to thrive
  - Squatting episodes
  - Cyanotic spells
  - Recurrent RTI.
- *Rule out pressure symptoms*
  - Dysphagia (esophagus)
  - Hoarseness of voice (recurrent laryngeal nerve)
  - Dyspnea (trachea).

Past History

- Similar illness
- HT, TB, DM and asthma
- IHD, CAD, MI (thrombolysis +/-).

Family History

- Similar h/o

- DM, TB, HT, IHD
- Parents marriage consanguineous.

Personal History

- Appetite
- Veg/Non-veg
- Bowel and bladder
- Alcohol ....amount.....duration
- Smoking.........nos........duration...
- Sleep.

Menstrual History

- Menarche.....LMP......
- Regular......amount....no(s) of pads used
- Associated pain.

Treatment History

Any history of penicillin prophylaxis.

GENERAL EXAMINATION

- Built and nourishment
- Conscious and cooperative
- Pallor, clubbing, edema,
- Cyanosis (Central/peripheral)
- Jaundice, lymphadenopathy

- Vital signs
  - Pulse—rate, rhythm
  - BP in right upper arm in supine position
  - Respiratory rate, type (thoracoabdominal)
  - Temperature (98.4°F).

CVS EXAMINATION

- Pulse: Rate, rhythm, volume, pulse deficit character, vessel wall, R-F delay, peripheral pulses
- BP in right upper arm in supine position
- JVP (Jugular venous pressure—is what we measure).

Inspection of Precordium

- Bony abnormality/spine
- Chest shape
- Trachea central
- Visible precordial bulge
- Visible pulsations
  - Apex (position)
  - Visible left sternal
  - Epigastric
  - Suprasternal.
- Scars, dilated veins, sinuses.

Palpation

- Apex—site, character
- Parasternal heave
- Palpable pulsation—epigastric, suprasternal, p2
- Other palpable sounds/thrills/pulsations in any other area of precordium
- Venous hum at base of neck.

Percussion

- Upper border liver (5th RICS in MCL)
- Liver span
- Right border of heart corresponds to right border of sternum
- Left border of heart corresponds to apex
- Percussion over 2nd left intercostal space.

Auscultation

- Mitral area
  - 2 sounds heard S1 and S2 (loud, normal, absent)
  - Murmurs
  - Other sounds.
- Tricuspid area
  - S1 and S2 normal
  - Murmurs
  - Other sounds.

- Aortic area
  - S1 and S2 normal (A_2 and P_2)
  - Murmurs
  - Other sounds.
- Pulmonary area
  - S1 and S2 normal (A_2 and P_2)
  - Murmurs
  - Other sounds.
- Splitting of S_2 (split paradoxical/normal)
- Carotid/femoral/renal bruit.

Murmur

- Grade, type, character—low/high pitch
- Radiation
- Best heard in which site/position
- With bell/diaphragm of stethoscope
- Breath held in expiration/inspiration
- Any presystolic accentuation
- Other sounds—opening snap, ejection click (if, any).

ABDOMEN EXAMINATION

- Hepatosplenomegaly, ascites
- Renal bruit.

RESPIRATORY EXAMINATION

- Normal vesicular breath sounds
- Adventitious sounds.

NERVOUS SYSTEM EXAMINATION

- Facial symmetry, reflexes
- Any neurological deficit.

DIAGNOSIS

- Sinus rhythm/irregular pulse
- Rheumatic/congenital heart disease
- Valvular lesion—MR, MS, AR, AS, PS, PR, TR, TS
- Pulmonary hypertension (2nd intercostal pulsation, palpable P2)
- Cardiac failure (↑ JVP, edema+, tender hepatomegaly)
- Infective endocarditis (fever, pallor, hematuria, splenomegaly).

Example

RHD with MS with pulmonary HT with no evidence of cardiac failure, in sinus rhythm and no evidence of infective endocarditis.

CHAPTER

5

Gastrointestinal System Case Proforma

Name ...., Age ...., Sex ....
Address ...., Occupation ....
Socioeconomic status ....
Date of admission..

PRESENTING COMPLAINT

....

....

HISTORY

History of Present Illness

- *Abdomen pain*
  - Onset, duration, progress, intensity
  - Site, type, radiation
  - Lasting, timing
  - Aggravating factors—food/vomiting
  - Relieving factors—drugs/food/flatus/posture/vomiting/defecation.

- *Abdomen distension*
  - Onset, duration, progress
  - Aggravating factors
  - Relieving factors—drugs/others.
- *Dysphagia*
  - Onset, duration, progress
  - Relating to solid/liquids
  - Aggravating factors
  - Relieving factors—drugs/others.
- *Vomiting*
  - Onset, duration, progress
  - Episodes, projectile, timing
  - Nausea
  - Aggravating factors
  - Relieving factors—drugs/food.
- *Vomitus*
  - Amount
  - Recent food
  - Color (bilious/blood stained)
  - Foul smelling.
- *Hematemesis*
  - Onset, duration, progress
  - Amount
  - Number of episodes

  - Color—bright red (fresh)/dark red (altered)
  - Mixed with food particles
  - Aggravating factors
  - Relieving factors.
- *Motion*
  - Amount, color, solid/watery
  - Blood stained/mucoid
  - Tenesmus
  - Foul smelling.
- *Melena (tarry black stools)*
  - Onset, duration, progress
  - Associated straining
  - Loose/semisolid
  - History of drugs, e.g. iron tablets.
- *Diarrhea/constipation*
  - Onset, duration, progress
  - Episodes, timing
  - Aggravating factors—pain/food
  - Relieving factors—drugs.
- *Edema*
  - Onset, duration, progress
  - Site, pitting/non-pitting
  - Aggravating factors (oliguria)
  - Relieving factors (drugs—diuretic).

- *Jaundice*
  - Onset, duration, progress
  - Urine/stool color
  - History of injections, drug abuse, blood transfusion
  - Aggravating factors/relieving factors
  - History of itching.
- *Bleeding per rectum*
  - Onset, duration, progress
  - Aggravating factors—constipation
  - Associated pain.
- *Fever*
  - Onset, duration, progress
  - Grade, chills/rigor
  - Diurnal variation, periodicity.
- *Oliguria*
  - Onset, duration, progress
  - Daily amount, urine color
  - Dysuria
  - Hematuria.
- *Burning sensation while micturation*
  - Onset, duration, progress
  - Aggravating factors,
  - Relieving factors.

- *Anorexia*
  - Duration, associated weight loss
  - Weight loss—how much
  - Bone tenderness
  - Bleeding—manifestations
  - Fatigue/weakness.

  (Weight loss, bone tenderness, bleeding, fatigue/weakness: Malignancy)

Nutritional History

Past History

- Similar illness
- History of TB, DM, HT, IHD, asthma, jaundice
- History of blood transfusion/any surgery
- History of malaria, kala azar, drug intake
- Leukemia, hemolytic crisis.

Family History

- Similar history
- History of DM, TB, HT, IHD
- History of malaria, syphilis, jaundice, asthma
- Consanguineous marriage of parents.

Personal History

- Appetite
- Veg/Non-veg

- Bowel and bladder
- Alcohol—amount, duration
- Smoking—no(s)/day, duration
- Sleep.

Menstrual History

- Menarche—LMP
- Regular/not, amount—no(s) of pads used
- Associated pain.

Treatment History

(Hospitalization, drugs, duration)

Allergic History

GENERAL EXAMINATION

- Built and nourishment
- Conscious and cooperative
- Pallor, clubbing, edema
- Cyanosis (central/peripheral)
- Jaundice, lymphadenopathy
- Signs of liver failure
  - Icterus
  - Parotid gland enlargement
  - Alopecia → axillary/pubic/chest
  - Spider nevi

  - Gynecomastia
  - Palmar erythema
  - Dupuytren's contracture
  - White nails
  - Flapping tremor
  - Testicular atrophy
  - Ascites
- Rule out TB
  - Low grade fever
  - Lymphadenopathy
- Rule out bleeding diathesis
  - Purpuric spots/petechiae
  - Bruising
  - Gum bleeding
  - Any tenderness.

Vital Signs

- Pulse—rate, rhythm, volume, character, vessel wall, R-F delay, peripheral pulses
- BP in right upper arm in supine position
- Respiration—rate, type (thoracoabdominal)
- Temperature (98.4°F)
- JVP.

EXAMINATION OF GASTROINTESTINAL SYSTEM

Mouth and Throat

- Oral cavity (hygiene)
- Gums, teeth
- Tongue:
  - Size—hypertrophy/atrophy
  - Surface—smooth/bald
  - Color—pale/normal
  - Ulcer(s)—describe.
- Tonsils.

Abdomen Proper

Inspection

- Shape
- Flanks
- All quadrant move equally with respiration
- Umbilicus—central and inverted/everted
- Visible scars, masses, dilated veins
- Visible pulsations
- Visible peristalsis.

Palpation

- Local rise of temperature, tenderness
- Guarding
- Rigidity
- Palpable bruit
- Rebound tenderness
- **Liver** — ____ cm below the coastal margin in right midclavicular line
  - Tenderness +/-
  - Edges, surface, consistency
  - Moves with respiration
  - Inability to insinuate finger between mass and costal margin.
- Abdominal girth
- Symphysioumbilical height
- Xphiumbilical height

} in case of ascites

- **Spleen** — ____ cm below the coastal margin along its long axis
  - Tenderness +/-
  - Edges (notched), surface, consistency
  - Moves with respiration
  - Inability to insinuate fingers between mass and costal margin
  - Renal angles.

Percussion

- Liver dullness in 5th RICS in midclavicular line
- Liver span
- Fluid thrill ++
- Shifting dullness
- Cardiac dullness preserved
- Knee elbow position—minimal fluid (Puddle's sign).

Auscultation

- Bowel sounds (heard/normal/not)
- Venous hum—portal flow obstruction
- Arterial bruit—aneurysm/atherosclerosis
- Spleen bruit—hemangioma
- Liver bruit—hepatoma
- Renal bruit—renal artery stenosis.

Inguinal Region

Inspection

- Swellings, scars, hernia(s).

Palpation

- Inguinal nodes
- Swelling(s)—describe
- Hernia(s)—describe.

PR Examination
CVS Examination
Respiratory Examination
Nervous System Examination

DIAGNOSIS

- Alcoholic/chronic liver disease
- Probably cirrhosis
- Evidence of portal hypertension (splenomegaly, dilated veins, hematuria)
- Evidence of ascites (fluid thrills, shifting dullness)
- Evidence of hepatic-encephalopathy (altered sensorium, flapping tremor, sleep rhythm disturbances, constructional apraxia).

CHAPTER

6

Nervous System Case Proforma

Name ...., Age ...., Sex ....
Address................, Occupation ....
Socioeconomic status ....
Date of admission ....
Patient is .... left/right handed
Informant ....
(In unconscious/patient with altered sensorium)

PRESENTING COMPLAINT

....
....

HISTORY

History of Present Illness

- ***Weakness***—onset, duration, progress
  - Upper limb—lifting arm, buttoning
  - Lower limb—climbing stairs, getting up
  - Total paralysis
  - Tone—history of stiffness of limbs.

- ***Wasting of muscles***—proximal/distal
- ***Incoordination of movements***
  - History of unsteadiness of gait
  - History of falling to one side (cerebellar)
  - History of incoordination in dark (sensory)
  - History of involuntary movements (rest/intentional).
- ***Sensory system***
  - History of tingling, numbness, root pain
  - History of diminished/absent hot and cold sensation during bathing.
- ***Sphincter disturbances***
  - Difficulty in micturition
  - Hesitancy
  - Incontinence (dribbling)
  - Bowel—constipation/incontinence
  - Difficulty in swallowing
  - Ejaculation.
- ***Cranial nerves***

I	Sensation of smell
II	Vision—distant, near, color
III, IV, VI	Double vision
V	Face—tingling/numbness/difficulty chewing

VII Facial—asymmetry, dribbling of saliva, difficulty drinking water
VIII Vertigo, deafness, tinnitus
IX Hoarseness of voice, dysphagia
X Nasal twang
XI Shrugging of shoulders, tilting of head
XII Difficulty—swallowing/talking/nasal regurgitation

- ***Higher functions***
  - Restlessness, dysarthria, dysphasia
  - Altered sensorium.
- ***Raised intracranial tension***
  - Headache
    - Onset, duration, progress
    - Site, severity, quality, timing
    - Aggravating factors
    - Relieving factors
    - Associated migraine.
  - Vomiting
    - Onset, duration, progress
    - Episodes, projectile, timing, nausea
    - Amount, recent food
    - Color (bilious/blood stained)
    - Foul smelling.

- Blurring of vision
- History of ear discharge
- History of root pain.

- ***Convulsions***
  - Onset and end, focal/generalized (associated fall)
  - Biting of tongue
  - Incontinence of bladder/bowel (during fit)
  - After symptoms—sleep, automatism, headache, paralysis
  - Subsequent mental paralysis
  - History of birth complications (injuries), ear discharge, similar attack in infancy, fever
  - Recent/remote head injury.
- ***Unconsciousness***
  - Onset, duration, progress
  - Age at first attack and second attack
  - Shortest/longest interval
  - Aura.
- ***Fever***
  - Onset, duration, progress
  - Grade, chills/rigor
  - Diurnal variation
  - Type intermittent/continuous
  - Night sweats.

- ***Chest pain*** *(associated with myocardial infarction)*
  - Onset, duration, progress
  - Site, type, radiation.
- ***Stroke/paralysis***
  - Premonitory symptoms before onset
  - How did it come on?
  - Progress—recovery/worsening
  - Associated vomiting (hemorrhage)
  - Blurring vision (hypertension)
  - Symptoms of heart disease (embolic)
  - Symptoms of DVT (embolic).
- ***Dizziness***
  - Onset, duration, progress
  - Intermittent/continuous
  - Any worsening by change in position
  - History of trauma/deafness.

Past History

- Similar, TB, DM, asthma, IHD/infective endocarditis, atrial fibrilation, vaccination.

Family History

- Similar history
- History of DM, TB, HT, IHD.

Personal History

- Appetite
- Veg/Non-veg
- Bowel/bladder
- Alcohol—amount, duration
- Smoking—no(s)/day, duration
- Sleep.

Menstrual History

- Menarche.....LMP......
- Regular, amount....no(s) of pads used
- Associated pain.

Treatment History

GENERAL EXAMINATION

- Built and nourishment, conscious and cooperative
- Pallor
- Cyanosis
- Clubbing
- Edema
- Jaundice
- Lymphadenopathy
- JVP

- Vital signs
  - Pulse—rate, rhythm, volume
  - BP in right upper arm in supine position
  - Respiration—rate, type (thoracoabdominal)
  - Temperature (98.4°F).
- Neurocutaneous markers (hypo/hyperpigmented areas, café-au-lait spots)
- Thickened nerves (if any).

NERVOUS SYSTEM EXAMINATION

Higher Functions (Dominant Hand)

- **C**—Consciousness (fully conscious, responds to verbal command/pain)
- **C**—Cooperative
- **O**—Orientation in—time, place, person
- **M**—Memory—recent/past
- **I**—Intelligence (some mathematical problems)
- **H**—Hallucinations
- **D**—Delusions
- **S**—Speech: Aphasia/dysarthria, articulation, fluency, comprehension, naming, reading, writing.

Cranial Nerves (Right and Left Separately)

I. Sensation of smell (right and left)
   - Smell of various substance like peppermint, asafetida.

II. Vision (right and left)
   - Acuity—distant and near vision
   - Color vision
   - Visual field.

III, IV and VI (right and left)
   - Palpaberal fissure—bilaterally equal/not
   - Ptosis, squint, nystagmus
   - Diplopia (near/distant)
   - Size and shape of pupil
   - Direct and consensual reflexes (cataract beware)
   - Pupillary—constriction, symmetry
   - Cardinal movements
   - Accommodation reflex
   - Ciliospinal reflex—Horner's syndrome.

IV. Trigeminal (right and left)
   - *Sensory*—sensation over face—touch/pain/temperature
   - *Motor*—muscles of mastication—clench the teeth, open the mouth, deviation of jaw
   - *Reflexes*
     - Corneal reflex } Afferent and
     - Conjuctival reflex } efferent
       (look up and away from you)
     - Jaw jerk.

VII. Facial (right and left)

- Sensation of taste—anterior 2/3 of tongue (pull out tongue with gauge)
- Eyebrow raising, wrinkling of forehead
- Eye closure (against and without resistance)
- Teeth showing (ask to smile)
- Whistling
- Blowing of cheek
- Nasolabial folds
- Platysma.

VIII. Vestibulocochlear (right and left)

- Vertigo, vomiting, tinnitus
- Hearing tests—wrist watch, Rinne's, Weber's
- Nystagmus—caloric test.

IX and X. (right and left)

- H/o aspiration, regurgitation, dysphagia
  Dysphagia → Liquids (central cause)
  Dysphagia → Solids (peripheral cause)
- Nasal twang
- Taste posterior 1/3 of tongue
- Movements of palate and uvula
- Gag reflex.

XI. Accessory (right and left)
- Trapezius and sternocledomastoid
  - Shrugging of shoulders against resistance
  - Tilting of head against resistance.

XII. Hypoglossal
- Deviation of tongue }
- Size of tongue } After protruding tongue
- Movements/wasting }
- Fasciculations ← With tongue inside the mouth.

Motor System

- Movements and strength
- Bulk of muscles
- Tone
- Gait
- Reflexes—superficial, deep and visceral
- Coordination of movements
- Involuntary movements.

- *Upper limb*
  - Abductor pollicis brevis
  - Opponens pollics, 1st dorsal interossei
  - Interossei and lumbricals and flexors, fingers
  - Flexors, extensors of wrist
  - Brachioradialis, biceps, triceps
  - Supraspinatus, deltoid, infraspinatus
  - Pectoralis, serratus anterior, latissmus dorsi.
- *Trunk and abdomen*
  - Babinski's rising up sign
  - Beevor's sign — T-10
  - Erector spinae and muscles of back
  - Diaphragm
  - Trapezius lower part (approx. shoulder blades).
- *Lower limb*
  - Intrinsic muscles of foot—claw foot
  - Flexors of toes and foot
  - Flexors and extensors of knee
  - Flexors and extensors of thigh
  - Adduction and abduction of thigh, rotation of thigh.

Reflexes

- *Superficial reflexes*
  - Corneal, conjunctival, palatal, pharyngeal
  - Abdominal
  - Cremasteric
  - Anal
  - Bulbocavernous
  - Plantar.
- *Deep reflexes*
  - Jaw jerk V.—pons—V.
  - Biceps C—5,6
  - Supinator C—5,6 radial N.
  - Inverted supinator C—5
  - Triceps C—6,7 radial N.
  - Knee L—2,3 femoral N.
  - Ankle S—1,2 tibial N.
  - Clonus
- *Visceral reflexes*
  - Swallowing reflex
  - Defecation reflex, micturition, sexual function.

Involuntary Movements

- Chorea, athetosis, hemibalism, tremor, fasciculations

Sensory System

- History of slipping away of slippers
- History of feel of walking over wool
- Touch (light), pain, temperature } Superficial
- anterolateral system } Superficial
- Tactile localization } Cortical
- Two-point discrimination } Cortical
- Stereognosis } Cortical
- Vibratory sense } Deep (posterior column)
- Sense of position } Deep (posterior column)
- Joint sense } Deep (posterior column)

Cerebellar Signs

- Dysmetria—finger-nose, finger-finger, heel-knee
- Walking in straight line
- Drunken gait
- Nystagmus—horizontal
- Dysarthria—scanning speech
- Hypotonia
- Dysdiadokinesia
- Rebound phenomenon
- Pendular knee jerk.

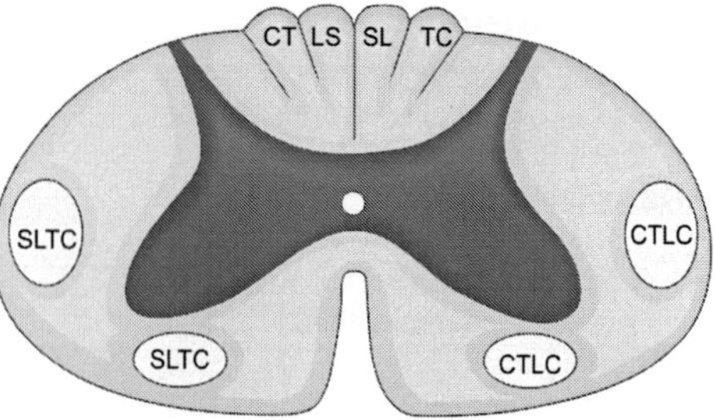

Signs of Meningeal Irritation

- Neck stiffness
- Kernig's sign
- Brudzinski sign.

Skull and Spine

- Shape, tenderness
- SLR—straight leg raising test
- Neck pain—cervical spondylitis.

Any Carotid Bruit

Any Thickening of Peripheral Nerves

CARDIOVASCULAR SYSTEM EXAMINATION

HT, AF, IHD, cardiomegaly, murmurs.

ABDOMEN EXAMINATION

Bladder.

DIAGNOSIS

(Disability + site + nature + etiology)

- Example 1:
  Known hypertensive now coming with CVA, left. hemiplegia, right/left facial nerve palsy having right/left-sided internal capsule lesion due to HT leading to hemorrhagic episode.
- Example 2:
  Quadriplegia, C-5, compressive, disc prolapse.

CHAPTER

7

Soft Skills

PROFESSIONAL ETIQUETTE AND ETIQUETTE TOWARD PATIENTS

- Look professional and be formal—patient will take you seriously
- Introduce yourself
- Take them into confidence
- Feel like being examined and respected, like we would expect from them if we were patient
- Be thankful to patient, they are doing a favor to us by being our subjects.

TIPS FOR CLINICAL EXAMINATIONS

- Wash your hands at beginning and end
- Introduce yourself to the patient
- Be polite
- Be thankful.

- Be gentle during an examination (remember the patient may have been examined 10 or 20 times before you). If the patient is in pain; cooperation will decrease.
- Remember patient rights:
  - Right to know everything
  - Right to comfort
  - Right to privacy
  - Right to know what's being done to them
  - Right to consent/refuse examination.

RESPIRATORY EXAMINATION, CARDIOVASCULAR (CVS) EXAMINATION, NEUROLOGICAL EXAMINATION

- Look professional
- Introduce yourself
- Be Polite, thankful and gentle
- Explain what the examination will entail—gain consent
- Wash hand
- Chaperone—respect the patient's dignity and privacy at all times
- Expose adequately
- Position patient.

- Post examination:
  - Thank the patient
  - Allow the patient to dress
  - Wash hands.

ABDOMINAL (GI) EXAMINATION

- Look professional
- Introduce yourself
- Be polite, thankful and gentle
- Explain what the examination will entail—gain consent
- Wash hand
- Chaperone
- Expose adequately
- Tender area to be examined last
- Ask examiner for examination of external genitalia and rectal examination—examiner may tell to skip
- Post examination
  - Allow the patient to dress
  - Say thanks
  - Wash hands.

BREAST EXAMINATION

As this is an intimate examination, it is pertinent to gain a good rapport with your patient, maintain good communication and ensure the patient's dignity at all times.

- Look professional
- Introduce yourself
- Be polite, thankful and gentle
- Explain what the examination will entail—gain consent
- Wash hand
- Chaperone—respect the patient's dignity and privacy at all times
- Expose adequately
- Position patient—initially sat on the edge of the bed
- Post examination:
  - Thank the patient
  - Allow the patient to dress
  - Wash hands.

THYROID EXAMINATION

- Look professional
- Introduce yourself
- Be polite, thankful and gentle
- Explain what the examination will entail—gain consent
- While doing above observe for:
  - Do they seem abnormally hyper- or hypo-active?
  - Do they appear sweaty?
  - What condition is their skin and hair?
  - Does their voice sound normal?
- Wash hand
- Expose adequately
- Post examination:
  - Thank the patient
  - Allow the patient to dress
  - Wash hands.

PREGNANT ABDOMEN EXAMINATION

This skill demonstrates two areas; your communication skills with the mother and your examination technique.

A few simple but friendly questions to help her gain your trust includes: "How are you feeling?", "Is this your first pregnancy?"

- Look professional
- Introduce yourself
- Be polite, thankful and gentle
- Explain what the examination will entail—gain consent
- Wash hand
- Expose adequately—ideally be exposed from the pubic bone to below her breasts
- Be gentle as your patient may have been examined many times before your turn
- Position patient: Patient should be lying on the bed, as flat as possible as per her comfort
- Post examination:
  - Thank the patient
  - Allow the patient to dress
  - Wash hands.

TESTICULAR EXAMINATION

- Look professional
- Introduce yourself
- Be polite, thankful and gentle
- Explain what the examination will entail—gain consent
- Wash hand
- Chaperone—respect the patient's dignity and privacy at all times
- Expose adequately—from the waist down, and with his shirt pulled up
- Patient position—standing
- Examiner should kneel down in front of and to the side of the patient, NOT directly in front of the patient
- Tender area to be examined last.
- Post examination:
  - Allow the patient to dress
  - Say thanks
  - Dispose of your gloves in applicable waste bin
  - Wash hands.

RECTAL (PR) EXAMINATION

- Look professional, introduce yourself
- Be polite, thankful and gentle
- Explain what the examination will entail—gain consent
- Wash hand
- Chaperone—respect the patient's dignity and privacy at all times
- Expose adequately—from the waist down, and with shirt pulled up
- Position patient
  - Lie on their left hand side
  - With their knees drawn up towards their chest
  - Their feet pushed forwards.
- Post examination:
  - Clean off any lubricant left around the anus
  - Allow the patient to dress
  - Thank the patient
  - Remove and dispose of your gloves in the clinical waste bin
  - Dispose of your gloves in applicable waste bin
  - Wash hands.